The Diet Detective: Uncovering the Truth About Popular Diets

By Randall Skyms

Introduction:

Welcome to "The Diet Detective: Uncovering the Truth About Popular Diets," a comprehensive guide to navigating the often-complicated world of nutrition and diet. This book is written by Randall Skyms, a world-renowned bodybuilder and certified strength and conditioning specialist who has been working with athletes for over a decade. With his extensive knowledge and experience, Randall provides readers with a unique perspective on the subject of diet and nutrition, offering insights into the latest scientific research and dispelling the many myths and misconceptions that surround the various diets that are currently popular.

Background:

For many years, Randall Skyms has been at the forefront of the fitness and health industry, working with some of the world's top athletes and helping them to achieve their goals and reach their full potential. Throughout his career, he has seen firsthand the impact that diet has on athletic performance, and he has become deeply passionate about helping people understand the importance of nutrition for their overall health and well-being.

In recent years, the world of diet and nutrition has become increasingly complex, with new fad diets appearing on a regular basis and conflicting nutritional claims being made by a range of experts and influencers. This has left many people feeling overwhelmed and unsure about what to eat and what to avoid. Randall realized that there was a real need for a comprehensive guide that could help people make sense of the many different diets that are available and provide them with the information they need to make informed decisions about their own health and nutrition.

Purpose of Writing the Book:

The purpose of "The Diet Detective: Uncovering the Truth About Popular Diets" is to provide readers with a clear and concise overview of the latest scientific research on diet and nutrition, and to help dispel the myths and misconceptions that surround the various diets that are currently popular. Through his extensive knowledge and experience, Randall offers a unique perspective on the subject, providing readers with insights into the latest findings and helping them to make sense of the often-confusing world of diet and nutrition.

The book covers a range of popular diets, from low-carb and ketogenic diets, to vegetarian and vegan diets, to gluten-free and paleo diets. Each chapter provides a detailed analysis of the scientific evidence behind each diet, including the potential benefits and drawbacks, and offering clear and practical advice for those who are considering following the diet.

In addition to providing readers with a comprehensive overview of the various diets, Randall also offers tips and advice for those who are looking to optimize their nutrition and lead a healthier lifestyle. He covers topics such as meal planning, portion control, and the importance of hydration, and provides a range of practical tools and resources that can help readers to achieve their goals.

Conclusion:

Whether you are an athlete looking to optimize your performance, or simply someone who wants to lead a healthier and more balanced lifestyle, "The Diet Detective: Uncovering the Truth About Popular Diets" is the ultimate resource for uncovering the truth about popular diets. With his extensive knowledge and experience, Randall provides readers with the information they need to make informed decisions about their own health and nutrition, and helps to dispel the many myths and misconceptions that surround the subject of diet and nutrition. This book is a must-read for anyone who is serious about their health and well-being, and who wants to take control of their diet and nutrition.

Table of Contents:

Chapter 1: Introduction to Popular Diets

This chapter provides an overview of the various diets that are currently popular, including low-carb, low-fat, vegan, paleo, Mediterranean, ketogenic, DASH, and intermittent fasting. It sets the stage for the rest of the book and provides readers with a background on the subject of diet and nutrition.

Chapter 2: The Low-Carb Diet

This chapter provides an in-depth analysis of the low-carb diet, including its history, the scientific evidence behind it, and the potential benefits and drawbacks of following this type of diet.

Chapter 3: The Low-Fat Diet

This chapter provides an in-depth analysis of the low-fat diet, including its history, the scientific evidence behind it, and the potential benefits and drawbacks of following this type of diet.

Chapter 4: The Vegan Diet

This chapter provides an in-depth analysis of the vegan diet, including its history, the scientific evidence behind it, and the potential benefits and drawbacks of following this type of diet.

Chapter 5: The Paleolithic Diet

This chapter provides an in-depth analysis of the paleo diet, including its history, the scientific evidence behind it, and the potential benefits and drawbacks of following this type of diet.

Chapter 6: The Mediterranean Diet

This chapter provides an in-depth analysis of the Mediterranean diet, including its history, the scientific evidence behind it, and the potential benefits and drawbacks of following this type of diet.

Chapter 7: The Ketogenic Diet

This chapter provides an in-depth analysis of the ketogenic diet, including its history, the scientific evidence behind it, and the potential benefits and drawbacks of following this type of diet.

Chapter 8: The DASH Diet

This chapter provides an in-depth analysis of the DASH diet, including its history, the scientific evidence behind it, and the potential benefits and drawbacks of following this type of diet.

Chapter 9: The Intermittent Fasting Diet

This chapter provides an in-depth analysis of the intermittent fasting diet, including its history, the scientific evidence behind it, and the potential benefits and drawbacks of following this type of diet.

Chapter 10: Evaluating the Effectiveness of Popular Diets

This chapter provides a comprehensive evaluation of the various popular diets, including the strengths and weaknesses of each one, and offering readers the information they need to make an informed decision about which diet is right for them.

Chapter 11: Understanding the Pros and Cons of Popular Diets

This chapter provides an in-depth analysis of the pros and cons of each of the popular diets, including the potential benefits and drawbacks, and helping readers to understand the impact of each diet on their overall health and well-being.

Chapter 12: Finding the Right Diet for You

This chapter provides practical advice for readers who are looking to find the right diet for them, including tips on how to assess their individual needs and goals, and how to choose the diet that is right for them.

Chapter 13: Creating a Sustainable and Balanced Diet

This chapter provides practical advice for readers who are looking to create a sustainable and balanced diet, including tips on how to plan and prepare healthy meals, and how to maintain a healthy and balanced diet over the long term.

Chapter 14: Overcoming Diet Fads and Quick Fixes

This chapter provides practical advice for readers who are looking to overcome the lure of fad diets and quick fixes, and provides strategies for maintaining a healthy and balanced diet over the long term.

Chapter 15: Staying Healthy and Achieving Your Diet Goals
This chapter provides practical advice for readers who are looking to stay healthy and achieve their diet goals, including tips on how to stay motivated, how to avoid common pitfalls, and how to maintain a healthy and balanced lifestyle over the long term. The chapter concludes by emphasizing the importance of a healthy and balanced diet, and encourages readers to take control of their health and well-being by making informed decisions about their diets.

Chapter 1: Introduction to Popular Diets

Diet and nutrition have become hot topics in recent years, with a wide variety of diets

being promoted as the best way to lose weight, improve health, and achieve wellness.

From low-carb diets that restrict carbohydrates, to low-fat diets that limit fat intake, to

vegan diets that eliminate animal products, there are many diets to choose from. Each of these diets claims to be the best, and each has its own unique set of benefits and drawbacks.

The purpose of this chapter is to provide an overview of the most popular diets, and to help readers understand the basics of each. This chapter will provide a brief description of each diet, as well as its key principles, benefits, and drawbacks. By the end of this chapter, readers will have a better understanding of the different types of diets that are currently popular, and will be in a better position to choose the right diet for their individual needs.

Low-Carb Diets

Low-carb diets are diets that restrict the intake of carbohydrates. The idea behind this type of diet is that carbohydrates are the main source of energy for the body, and by restricting carbohydrates, the body is forced to burn fat for fuel instead. This process is known as ketosis, and it is believed to lead to weight loss, improved energy levels, and a reduction in hunger and cravings.

The most well-known low-carb diet is the Atkins diet, which was created in the 1970s by Dr. Robert Atkins. The Atkins diet is a four-phase diet that starts with a strict induction phase, in which carbohydrates are restricted to just 20 grams per day. The diet then gradually increases the amount of carbohydrates allowed, with the goal being to find the individual's "carbohydrate tolerance" and maintain that level for life.

Low-Fat Diets

Low-fat diets are diets that restrict the intake of fat. The idea behind this type of diet is that fat is a source of calories, and by reducing the amount of fat in the diet, the body is able to lose weight. Low-fat diets are typically high in carbohydrates, and they are often recommended for people who are looking to lose weight, lower their cholesterol levels, or improve their heart health.

The most well-known low-fat diet is the Ornish diet, which was created by Dr. Dean Ornish in the 1980s. The Ornish diet is a low-fat, plant-based diet that restricts the intake of animal products and emphasizes the consumption of fruits, vegetables, whole grains, and legumes.

Vegan Diets

Vegan diets are diets that eliminate all animal products, including meat, poultry, fish, dairy, and eggs. The idea behind this type of diet is that animal products are harmful to the body, and that a diet based solely on plant-based foods is healthier. Vegan diets are typically high in carbohydrates, and they are often recommended for people who are looking to improve their overall health, reduce their risk of chronic disease, or protect the environment.

The most well-known vegan diet is the Engine 2 diet, which was created by Rip Esselstyn in the 2000s. The Engine 2 diet is a low-fat, plant-based diet that emphasizes the consumption of whole, unprocessed foods and restricts the intake of processed foods and added sugars.

Paleolithic Diets

Paleolithic diets are diets that are based on the foods that were consumed by our ancestors during the Paleolithic era. The idea behind this type of diet is that our bodies are genetically adapted to the foods that were consumed during this time, and that a diet based on these foods is healthier for us than a diet based on the processed and highly refined foods that are commonly consumed today. Paleolithic diets are typically high in protein and fat, and they emphasize the consumption of meat, poultry, fish, vegetables, fruits, and nuts.

The most well-known paleolithic diet is the Paleolithic diet, also known as the "caveman diet." This diet is based on the principles of the Paleolithic era, and it restricts the intake of grains, legumes, dairy products, and added sugars. Instead, it emphasizes the consumption of meat, poultry, fish, vegetables, fruits, and nuts.

Mediterranean Diets

Mediterranean diets are diets that are based on the traditional eating patterns of people living in the Mediterranean region. The idea behind this type of diet is that the Mediterranean way of eating is associated with good health and a reduced risk of chronic disease. Mediterranean diets are typically high in carbohydrates, and they emphasize the consumption of olive oil, nuts, fruits, vegetables, and legumes.

The most well-known Mediterranean diet is the Mediterranean diet, which is based on the traditional eating patterns of people living in the Mediterranean region. This diet emphasizes the consumption of olive oil, nuts, fruits, vegetables, and legumes, and it restricts the intake of meat and dairy products.

Ketogenic Diets

Ketogenic diets are diets that are high in fat, moderate in protein, and low in carbohydrates. The idea behind this type of diet is that by restricting carbohydrates and consuming high amounts of fat, the body is able to enter a state of ketosis, in which it burns fat for fuel instead of carbohydrates. This process is believed to lead to weight loss, improved energy levels, and a reduction in hunger and cravings.

The most well-known ketogenic diet is the ketogenic diet, which was originally developed in the 1920s to treat epilepsy. This diet is a high-fat, moderate-protein, low-carbohydrate diet that restricts the intake of carbohydrates and emphasizes the consumption of fats and proteins.

DASH Diets

DASH diets are diets that are designed to lower blood pressure. The acronym DASH stands for Dietary Approaches to Stop Hypertension, and these diets are high in fruits, vegetables, whole grains, and low-fat dairy products, and they are low in sodium, saturated and total fat, and added sugars. The idea behind this type of diet is that by reducing sodium and increasing potassium intake, blood pressure can be lowered, reducing the risk of heart disease and stroke.

The most well-known DASH diet is the DASH diet, which was developed by the National Heart, Lung, and Blood Institute. This diet is a high-carbohydrate, low-fat diet that emphasizes the consumption of fruits, vegetables, whole grains, and low-fat dairy products, and it restricts the intake of sodium, saturated and total fat, and added sugars.

Intermittent Fasting Diets

Intermittent fasting diets are diets that alternate periods of fasting and eating. The idea behind this type of diet is that by restricting the number of hours in which food is consumed, the body is able to burn fat for fuel instead of carbohydrates. Intermittent fasting diets can be structured in a variety of ways, including daily fasts, alternate-day fasts, or fasting for several hours each day.

The most well-known intermittent fasting diet is the 16:8 diet, which involves fasting for 16 hours each day and eating during an 8-hour window. This diet is based on the idea that by restricting the number of hours in which food is consumed, the body is able to burn fat for fuel instead of carbohydrates.

Chapter 2: The Low-Carb Diet

The low-carb diet is one of the most popular diets in recent history. It has been used by millions of people as a means of losing weight, improving health, and increasing athletic performance. In this chapter, we will take a closer look at what exactly the low-carb diet is, where it comes from, and the science behind it.

A Brief History of the Low-Carb Diet

The idea of a low-carb diet is not a new one. For centuries, humans have been eating diets that are low in carbohydrates and high in protein and fat. In the late 19th and early 20th centuries, the popularity of low-carb diets increased due to the popularity of the "Banting" diet, which was named after William Banting, an English man who wrote a popular pamphlet about his success in losing weight on a low-carb diet.

However, it wasn't until the 1990s that the low-carb diet really took off. This was due in part to the publication of Dr. Robert Atkins' book "Dr. Atkins' Diet Revolution", which popularized the idea of a low-carb diet for weight loss. Since then, the low-carb diet has become one of the most popular diets in the world, with millions of people following it in one form or another.

The Science Behind the Low-Carb Diet

The underlying idea behind the low-carb diet is that carbohydrates are the primary cause of weight gain and other health problems. When we eat carbohydrates, they are broken down into glucose, which is then used as energy by the body. However, when we eat more carbohydrates than our bodies need for energy, the excess glucose is stored as fat.

By reducing the amount of carbohydrates in our diets, we can reduce the amount of glucose that is stored as fat, leading to weight loss. Additionally, by reducing the amount of glucose in our diets, we can also reduce insulin resistance, which is a major factor in the development of many chronic diseases such as type 2 diabetes, heart disease, and cancer.

The Benefits of the Low-Carb Diet

There are a number of benefits to following a low-carb diet, including:

1. Weight loss: One of the most well-known benefits of the low-carb diet is weight loss. By reducing the amount of carbohydrates in your diet, you can reduce the amount of glucose that is stored as fat, leading to weight loss.
2. Improved insulin sensitivity: As mentioned above, reducing the amount of glucose in your diet can also reduce insulin resistance, leading to improved insulin sensitivity and a reduced risk of developing chronic diseases such as type 2 diabetes.
3. Increased energy: Many people who follow the low-carb diet report increased energy levels, as their bodies are able to use fat for energy instead of relying on carbohydrates.
4. Improved mental clarity: Some people also report improved mental clarity and focus on a low-carb diet, as the brain is able to use ketones for energy instead of glucose.

The Drawbacks of the Low-Carb Diet

While there are many benefits to the low-carb diet, there are also some drawbacks to consider. These include:

1. Difficult to follow: The low-carb diet can be difficult to follow, especially for those who are used to eating a diet that is high in carbohydrates. It can also be difficult to stick to the diet in social situations, as many popular foods contain high amounts of carbohydrates.

2. Risk of nutrient deficiencies: By limiting the amount of carbohydrates in your diet, you may also be limiting your intake of important

Chapter 3: The Low-Fat Diet

The low-fat diet has been one of the most popular diets in recent decades, with many people turning to this diet as a way to lose weight and improve their health. This chapter provides an in-depth examination of the low-fat diet, including its history, the scientific evidence behind it, and the potential benefits and drawbacks of following this type of diet.

The low-fat diet originated in the late 1970s and early 1980s as a response to the growing obesity epidemic and concerns about the role of fat in heart disease. At the time, the prevailing wisdom was that a diet high in fat was one of the primary causes of heart disease, and that reducing the amount of fat in the diet would help to prevent this disease. This led to a widespread movement towards low-fat diets, with many people replacing high-fat foods with low-fat and fat-free products.

In recent years, however, the scientific evidence behind the low-fat diet has come under scrutiny, with some studies suggesting that it may not be as effective as once thought. One of the main criticisms of the low-fat diet is that it does not take into account the type of fat that is being consumed. While some types of fat, such as trans fats and saturated fats, have been linked to negative health effects, other types of fat, such as monounsaturated and polyunsaturated fats, are considered to be healthy and may actually have beneficial effects on heart health.

In addition to this, some studies have found that low-fat diets may not be as effective for weight loss as other types of diets. This may be due to the fact that many low-fat products are high in added sugars and carbohydrates, which can lead to an increase in calories and weight gain. Some studies have also found that low-fat diets may not be as effective for improving cholesterol levels and heart health as other types of diets, such as the Mediterranean diet.

Despite these criticisms, the low-fat diet still has its proponents, who argue that it can be an effective way to improve health and prevent chronic diseases. One of the key benefits of the low-fat diet is that it is often low in calories, which can help people to lose weight. In addition, many low-fat products are also low in saturated fat, which has been linked to an increased risk of heart disease.

One of the biggest challenges of following the low-fat diet is that it can be difficult to stick to, as many people find it difficult to give up high-fat foods. In addition, many low-fat products are not as flavorful or satisfying as their high-fat counterparts, which can make it difficult to stick to the diet in the long term.

In conclusion, the low-fat diet has been a popular diet for many years, but the scientific evidence behind it has come under scrutiny in recent years. While there are potential benefits to following a low-fat diet, such as reducing calories and reducing the intake of saturated fat, there are also drawbacks, such as the potential to increase the intake of added sugars and carbohydrates. Ultimately, the best diet for any individual will depend on their individual needs and goals, and it is important to consult with a healthcare provider or registered dietitian before making any changes to your diet.

Chapter 4: The Vegan Diet

The vegan diet has gained a significant amount of popularity in recent years, with millions of people around the world choosing to follow this type of diet for both ethical and health reasons. In this chapter, we will provide an in-depth analysis of the vegan diet, including its history, the scientific evidence behind it, and the potential benefits and drawbacks of following this type of diet.

The history of the vegan diet can be traced back to ancient civilizations, such as ancient Greece and India, where vegetarianism was practiced for both ethical and health reasons. However, the modern-day vegan movement was formed in the 19th century by a group of British vegetarians who advocated for the elimination of animal products from the human diet. This movement gained momentum over the years, and today, veganism has become a widely recognized lifestyle choice. The number of vegans in the world has grown rapidly, and there are now numerous vegan options available in grocery stores, restaurants, and other food establishments.

The vegan diet is based on the belief that it is possible to meet all of our nutritional needs through plant-based foods, and that animal products are not necessary for good health. This type of diet excludes all animal products, including meat, dairy, eggs, and honey. The scientific evidence behind the vegan diet is mixed. On one hand, a well-planned vegan diet can provide all the essential nutrients our bodies need, including protein, iron, calcium, and vitamins B12 and D. Plant-based foods are also high in fiber, antioxidants, and phytochemicals, which have been shown to have numerous health benefits. For example, a diet rich in fruits, vegetables, whole grains, and legumes has been shown to reduce the risk of heart disease, stroke, and certain types of cancer.

However, following a vegan diet can also have some drawbacks. One of the biggest concerns is the risk of nutrient deficiencies, particularly with regards to vitamin B12, iron, and calcium. These nutrients are primarily found in animal products and are essential for good health. If not obtained from other sources, a deficiency in these nutrients can lead to a number of health problems, such as anemia, nervous system damage, and osteoporosis. For this reason, it is important for individuals following a vegan diet to be mindful of their nutrient intake and to take steps to ensure that their needs are met through other sources, such as fortified foods or dietary supplements.

In conclusion, the vegan diet has both potential benefits and drawbacks, and it is important for individuals to be aware of both when making the decision to follow this type of diet. A well-planned vegan diet can provide all the essential nutrients our bodies need and has been shown to have numerous health benefits. However, it is also important to be mindful of potential nutrient deficiencies and to take steps to ensure that these needs are met through other sources. Individuals who are considering following a vegan diet should consult with a healthcare provider or a registered dietitian to ensure that they are able to meet their nutritional needs in a safe and healthy manner.

The next chapter will continue our exploration of popular diets by examining the paleolithic diet, which has gained popularity in recent years for its potential health benefits and simplicity. As with any diet, it is important to be mindful of both the potential benefits and drawbacks, and to make informed decisions based on individual needs and goals.

Chapter 5: The Paleolithic Diet

The Paleolithic diet, also known as the "caveman diet," is based on the idea that humans should eat the same way our ancestors did during the Paleolithic era, when we were hunters and gatherers. This era lasted from 2.5 million to 10,000 years ago, and it is believed that our bodies have not evolved to adapt to the modern Western diet, which is high in processed foods and refined sugars. The paleo diet aims to correct this mismatch by returning to a diet that is more in line with our ancestral heritage.

The paleo diet is based on the following principles:

- Consume a diet that is high in protein and healthy fats, such as those found in fish, grass-fed beef, eggs, and avocados.
- Avoid processed foods, refined sugars, and unhealthy fats, such as those found in vegetable oils and processed snacks.
- Eat plenty of fruits, vegetables, and nuts.
- Eliminate grains, legumes, and dairy, which are believed to have been introduced into the human diet relatively recently.

The paleo diet has gained popularity in recent years as a way to improve health and lose weight. Proponents of the paleo diet argue that it can help improve energy levels, reduce inflammation, and prevent chronic diseases such as heart disease, type 2 diabetes, and certain cancers. They also claim that the paleo diet can help people lose weight by reducing caloric intake, as well as by promoting a more balanced and healthy relationship with food.

However, there is limited scientific evidence to support the benefits of the paleo diet, and some experts believe that it may be too restrictive and nutritionally inadequate. For example, eliminating grains, legumes, and dairy from the diet can lead to a deficiency in essential nutrients such as fiber, calcium, and B vitamins. Additionally, relying heavily on meat and animal products can increase the risk of heart disease and other health problems.

In conclusion, the paleo diet may be a useful tool for some people to improve their health and reach their weight loss goals. However, it is important to approach this diet

with caution, as it may not be suitable for everyone and can have potential health risks.
It is also important to consult with a doctor or a registered dietitian before starting any
new diet, especially if you have a history of health problems or are taking medication.

In the next chapter, we will explore another popular diet, the Mediterranean diet, which
is based on the traditional eating patterns of the people living along the Mediterranean
Sea. This diet has been associated with numerous health benefits, and has been shown
to help prevent chronic diseases and promote longevity.

Chapter 6: The Mediterranean Diet

The Mediterranean Diet is a style of eating that is based on the traditional dietary habits
of the people living in the Mediterranean region, particularly Greece and Italy, in the

mid-20th century. This way of eating is characterized by a high intake of fruits, vegetables, whole grains, legumes, nuts, and seeds, as well as a moderate intake of fish and poultry, and a low intake of red meat, dairy products, and processed foods. The use of olive oil as the primary source of fat is also a hallmark of the Mediterranean diet.

The origins of the Mediterranean diet can be traced back to the rural populations of Greece and Italy, where people relied on local, seasonal ingredients to nourish themselves. Over time, this way of eating was adopted and modified by other Mediterranean countries, and it became a cultural tradition that was passed down from generation to generation. Today, the Mediterranean diet is considered to be one of the healthiest dietary patterns in the world, and it is often recommended by health professionals as a means of reducing the risk of chronic diseases such as heart disease, type 2 diabetes, and certain types of cancer.

One of the key components of the Mediterranean diet is its emphasis on whole, minimally processed foods. By consuming a wide variety of fruits, vegetables, whole grains, and legumes, individuals following this diet can benefit from a wide range of vitamins, minerals, and antioxidants that are essential for good health. Additionally, the moderate consumption of fish and poultry, along with the low consumption of red meat, dairy products, and processed foods, can help to reduce the risk of heart disease and other chronic health conditions.

Another key aspect of the Mediterranean diet is the use of olive oil as the primary source of fat. Olive oil is a monounsaturated fat that has been shown to have a number of health benefits, including reducing inflammation and improving heart health. In fact, several studies have demonstrated that people who follow a Mediterranean diet that is rich in olive oil are less likely to develop heart disease and other chronic health conditions.

Despite its many potential benefits, the Mediterranean diet is not without its drawbacks. For one, it can be difficult to follow for people who are used to eating a Western-style diet that is high in processed foods and unhealthy fats. Additionally, the cost of following this diet can be a barrier for some individuals, particularly those who live in areas where whole, minimally processed foods are not readily available or are more expensive.

In conclusion, the Mediterranean diet is a healthy and balanced way of eating that has been shown to have a number of benefits for both physical and mental health. By focusing on whole, minimally processed foods and using olive oil as the primary source of fat, individuals following this diet can improve their overall health and reduce their risk of developing chronic health conditions. However, it is important to remember that no diet is perfect, and that finding the right diet for you may require some trial and error. In the next chapter, we will examine the ketogenic diet, another popular dietary pattern that has gained a lot of attention in recent years.

Chapter 7: The Ketogenic Diet

The ketogenic diet, also known as the "keto diet", has gained significant popularity in recent years, particularly for its potential to promote weight loss and improve health markers such as blood sugar and cholesterol levels. This high-fat, low-carbohydrate diet has been around for nearly a century, initially developed as a treatment for epilepsy in children. However, in recent years, it has become a popular weight loss and wellness trend, with many proponents claiming that it can help people lose weight, improve their energy levels, and even treat a range of chronic conditions.

The ketogenic diet is based on the premise that reducing carbohydrate intake forces the body to burn fat for energy instead of glucose, leading to a state of ketosis. During this metabolic state, the liver produces ketones, which become the primary fuel source for the body. The diet typically consists of high-fat foods such as meat, poultry, fish, eggs, dairy products, and healthy oils, along with low-carb vegetables such as spinach, broccoli, and kale. It also restricts high-carbohydrate foods such as bread, pasta, and sugar.

The scientific evidence behind the ketogenic diet is mixed. Some studies have shown that it can be effective for weight loss and improving certain health markers, such as reducing inflammation, improving insulin sensitivity, and lowering blood sugar levels. However, other studies have found that it may have negative effects on heart health, cholesterol levels, and gut health. Additionally, the long-term effects of the diet are not well understood and it can be difficult to follow for many people, particularly due to its strict limitations on carbohydrates.

One example of the potential benefits of the ketogenic diet is a study published in the journal Diabetes Therapy, which found that a low-carb, high-fat diet was more effective for weight loss and improving glycemic control in people with type 2 diabetes than a low-fat, high-carb diet. Another study, published in the journal Nutritional Neuroscience, found that a ketogenic diet improved memory and cognitive function in older adults.

However, it's important to note that not all experts agree on the benefits of the ketogenic diet. Some argue that it may have negative effects on heart health, as it can increase cholesterol levels and the risk of heart disease. Additionally, the diet can be difficult to follow for many people, particularly due to its strict limitations on carbohydrates, and can lead to nutritional deficiencies if not properly balanced with enough fiber, vitamins, and minerals.

In conclusion, while the ketogenic diet may have potential benefits for weight loss and improving certain health markers, it is important to consider the potential drawbacks and to talk to a healthcare professional before starting any new diet. As with any diet, it is important to focus on a balanced and sustainable approach that meets your individual needs and helps you achieve your health goals in the long-term.

Chapter 8: The DASH Diet

The DASH diet, which stands for Dietary Approaches to Stop Hypertension, is a dietary pattern that is designed to help lower blood pressure levels. This diet was developed in response to the growing problem of high blood pressure in the United States, and it has since become one of the most widely recommended dietary patterns for people with this condition. The DASH diet is also highly recommended for people looking to improve their overall health and prevent a range of chronic diseases, including heart disease, stroke, and type 2 diabetes.

The main principles of the DASH diet are centered around consuming a variety of nutrient-dense foods, including plenty of fruits and vegetables, whole grains, lean proteins, and low-fat dairy products. The diet also restricts the intake of added sugars, saturated fats, and sodium, which are known to have negative effects on health. By following these guidelines, the DASH diet aims to reduce the risk of hypertension and improve overall health.

One of the key strengths of the DASH diet is that it is backed by a large body of scientific evidence. Numerous studies have shown that the DASH diet is effective in reducing blood pressure levels, and some studies have even shown that it can lower blood pressure levels to a similar extent as some medications. Additionally, the DASH diet has been shown to have positive effects on other markers of health, including cholesterol levels, blood sugar control, and body weight.

However, like any diet, the DASH diet also has some potential drawbacks. One of the main criticisms of the diet is that it can be difficult to follow, especially for people who are used to eating a lot of processed foods and high amounts of sodium. Additionally, some people may find the restrictions on certain foods, such as added sugars and saturated fats, to be challenging.

Despite these drawbacks, the DASH diet remains one of the most widely recommended diets for people with high blood pressure and those looking to improve their overall health. This is because it provides a balanced and nutritionally complete diet that is rich in a range of essential vitamins and minerals, and it is also relatively easy to follow for those who are willing to make the necessary changes to their eating habits.

In conclusion, the DASH diet is a highly effective diet that is designed to help lower blood pressure levels and improve overall health. While there may be some challenges associated with following this type of diet, the potential benefits, including reduced risk of hypertension, improved cholesterol levels, and better blood sugar control, make it an excellent choice for people looking to improve their health and prevent chronic diseases. In the next chapter, we will take a closer look at the Intermittent Fasting diet, which has become increasingly popular in recent years.

Chapter 9: The Intermittent Fasting Diet

In this chapter, we will delve into the world of intermittent fasting, exploring its origins, scientific evidence, and the potential benefits and drawbacks of following this type of diet. Intermittent fasting is a pattern of eating where periods of eating are alternated with periods of fasting. The most popular forms of intermittent fasting include time-restricted eating and alternate-day fasting.

For example, with time-restricted eating, an individual may only eat during a specific window of time, such as 12pm to 8pm, and fast the rest of the day. With alternate-day fasting, an individual alternates between eating and fasting every other day.

The benefits of intermittent fasting include improved insulin sensitivity, reduced inflammation, and potential weight loss. However, there are also potential drawbacks, such as the possibility of overeating during eating periods and potential nutrient deficiencies.

It is important to remember that everyone is unique and what works for one person may not work for another. Intermittent fasting is a form of dieting that requires careful consideration and monitoring, as it is not suitable for everyone, particularly those with medical conditions or who are pregnant or breastfeeding.

In this chapter, we will take an in-depth look at the science behind intermittent fasting, examining the latest research and data to help readers make informed decisions about whether this type of diet is right for them.

Chapter 10: Evaluating the Effectiveness of Popular Diets

With so many different diets available today, it can be difficult to determine which one is right for you. This chapter aims to provide a comprehensive evaluation of the various popular diets, including the low-carb, low-fat, vegan, paleo, Mediterranean, ketogenic, DASH, and intermittent fasting diets. By understanding the strengths and weaknesses of each of these diets, you can make an informed decision about which one is right for you.

To begin, let's take a closer look at the low-carb diet. The low-carb diet has been around for decades and is based on the idea that reducing carbohydrate intake can help you lose weight and improve your overall health. While there is some evidence to support the effectiveness of this diet, it is important to keep in mind that it is not appropriate for everyone. For example, individuals who are diabetic or have kidney disease may need to limit their intake of certain types of carbohydrates, but may not need to follow a low-carb diet.

Next, let's examine the low-fat diet. This diet is based on the idea that reducing the amount of fat in your diet can help you lose weight and improve your overall health. However, recent research has called into question the effectiveness of this diet and has shown that a diet high in healthy fats, such as those found in olive oil and nuts, can actually be beneficial for weight loss and overall health.

The vegan diet is another popular option, and is based on the idea that consuming a plant-based diet can help improve your health and reduce your risk of certain diseases. While there is some evidence to support the benefits of this diet, it can be challenging to get all of the nutrients you need without consuming animal products. Additionally, people who follow a vegan diet must be mindful of their protein intake, as plant-based sources of protein may not be as complete as animal-based sources.

The paleo diet is based on the idea that our ancestors ate a diet high in protein and low in carbohydrates, and that this type of diet is ideal for human health. While there is some evidence to support the benefits of this diet, it can be challenging to follow in a modern, fast-paced world. Additionally, the paleo diet may not be appropriate for individuals who are lactose intolerant or have other dietary restrictions.

The Mediterranean diet is a well-balanced diet that is high in healthy fats, fruits, and vegetables, and low in red meat and dairy products. This diet has been shown to have numerous health benefits, including reducing the risk of heart disease, stroke, and certain types of cancer. However, it is important to keep in mind that this diet is not necessarily a weight loss diet, and may not be appropriate for individuals who need to limit their intake of certain types of fat.

The ketogenic diet is a high-fat, low-carbohydrate diet that is designed to put your body into a state of ketosis, where it burns fat for energy instead of carbohydrates. While this diet can be effective for weight loss, it can also be challenging to follow, and may not be appropriate for individuals who are diabetic or have kidney disease.

The DASH diet is a well-balanced diet that is designed to help lower blood pressure and reduce the risk of heart disease. This diet is high in fruits, vegetables, whole grains, and lean protein, and low in sodium and added sugars. While this diet can be effective for reducing blood pressure, it may not be appropriate for individuals who need to limit their intake of certain types of carbohydrates or who have other dietary restrictions.

Finally, this chapter concludes by discussing the importance of individualized approaches to diet and nutrition, as what works well for one person may not work as well for another. It is crucial to consider one's own unique needs and preferences, as well as to consult with a healthcare professional, when making decisions about which diet to follow. Ultimately, it is not just about finding the right diet, but also about developing a healthy and sustainable relationship with food and nourishing the body in a way that promotes overall well-being. The chapter ends by highlighting the key takeaways from the evaluations of popular diets and emphasizing the importance of finding the right balance in order to achieve and maintain optimal health.

Chapter 11: Understanding the Pros and Cons of Popular Diets

The vegan diet has been touted for its health benefits, including a lower risk of chronic diseases and a healthier gut microbiome. However, it can also be challenging to get all of the necessary nutrients, particularly protein and certain vitamins and minerals, without supplementing or carefully planning one's diet.

The paleo diet, which emphasizes the consumption of whole, minimally processed foods, can lead to improved gut health, weight loss, and reduced inflammation. However, it can also be restrictive and may lead to deficiencies in certain nutrients, such as calcium and vitamin D, if not properly balanced.

The Mediterranean diet, with its emphasis on fresh fruits and vegetables, whole grains, and healthy fats, has been linked to a lower risk of heart disease, cancer, and other chronic conditions. However, it may not be suitable for everyone and can be challenging to follow in certain cultural and financial contexts.

The ketogenic diet, which restricts carbohydrates and emphasizes the consumption of high-fat, low-carb foods, has been shown to be effective for weight loss and reducing the risk of certain chronic diseases. However, it can be difficult to follow long-term and may lead to nutrient deficiencies and digestive issues if not properly balanced.

The DASH diet, which emphasizes the consumption of whole, minimally processed foods and is low in salt, has been linked to a reduction in blood pressure and a lower risk of heart disease. However, it may be challenging to follow for some people and can be restrictive in certain cultural and financial contexts.

Intermittent fasting, which involves alternating periods of fasting with periods of eating, has been shown to be effective for weight loss, improving markers of heart health, and reducing the risk of certain chronic diseases. However, it may not be suitable for everyone and can be challenging to stick to, particularly for those with a history of disordered eating or those with certain medical conditions.

By understanding the pros and cons of each of these popular diets, readers can make an informed decision about which diet is right for them and their individual needs and goals.

Chapter 12: Finding the Right Diet for You

One of the biggest challenges when it comes to diet and nutrition is finding the right approach that works for you. With so many popular diets to choose from, it can be difficult to know where to start and what is best for your individual needs and goals.

The first step in finding the right diet for you is to assess your individual needs and goals. This may include considering factors such as your age, gender, activity level, health status, and any medical conditions you may have. For example, a low-carb diet may not be the best choice for someone with diabetes, while a high-protein diet may not be suitable for someone with kidney disease.

Once you have assessed your individual needs and goals, it is important to consider your personal preferences and lifestyle. This includes taking into account factors such as your cooking skills, food preferences, and the amount of time and effort you are willing to put into meal planning and preparation.

When it comes to choosing a diet, it is also important to consider the level of sustainability and balance. Some diets may be more restrictive or require more effort than others, making it difficult to stick to them over the long term. In addition, some diets may be more likely to result in nutrient deficiencies, while others may be overly focused on one particular type of food or macronutrient, leading to an unbalanced diet.

Once you have taken all of these factors into account, it is time to start exploring the different popular diets and determining which one is right for you. Here are a few tips to help you in your journey:

1. Educate yourself about each diet: Before making a decision, it is important to educate yourself about each diet and what it entails. This may include reading books, articles, and research studies, as well as consulting with a healthcare provider or registered dietitian.

2. Try it out: If you are unsure about a particular diet, consider giving it a try for a set period of time to see how it works for you. This can help you determine if the diet is sustainable, and if it results in any changes in your health, weight, or well-being.

3. Listen to your body: Ultimately, the most important factor in determining the right diet for you is listening to your body and how it responds. If you experience any negative side effects, such as fatigue, headaches, or digestive issues, it may be time to re-evaluate your diet and make adjustments as needed.

In conclusion, finding the right diet for you is a personal and individual journey that requires careful consideration of your needs, goals, preferences, and lifestyle. By taking the time to assess these factors and educate yourself about each of the popular diets, you can make an informed decision about which diet is right for you and ensure that you are able to maintain a healthy and balanced diet over the long term.

This chapter concludes with the importance of finding a diet that is sustainable and balanced, and how this is key to maintaining good health and well-being over the long term. By considering the various factors involved and taking a personalized approach, readers can find the diet that is right for them and achieve their health and wellness goals.

Chapter 13: Creating a Sustainable and Balanced Diet

The goal of creating a sustainable and balanced diet is to ensure that your body is receiving the necessary nutrients it needs to function optimally, while also satisfying your taste buds and avoiding the pitfalls of restrictive diets. In this chapter, we will provide practical advice for readers who are looking to create a sustainable and balanced diet, including tips on how to plan and prepare healthy meals, and how to maintain a healthy and balanced diet over the long term.

Planning and Preparing Healthy Meals

One of the keys to success in creating a sustainable and balanced diet is meal planning. This involves taking the time to plan out your meals for the week in advance, including breakfast, lunch, dinner, and snacks. This will not only help you to stick to your diet, but it will also save you time and money.

When planning your meals, it's important to consider the following:

- Eating a variety of nutrient-dense foods, such as fruits, vegetables, whole grains, lean proteins, and healthy fats.
- Balancing your meals so that they include a source of carbohydrates, protein, and healthy fats.

- Making sure to include at least one serving of fruit and one serving of vegetables in each meal.

- Incorporating healthy snacks, such as raw veggies and hummus, fruit, or a handful of nuts, into your daily routine.

Once you have your meal plan in place, it's time to start preparing your meals. To save time and make meal preparation easier, you can do the following:

- Cook in bulk and freeze leftovers for future meals.

- Use a slow cooker or instant pot to prepare meals in advance.

- Prep fruits and veggies ahead of time so they're ready to grab and go.

- Make healthy snacks, such as trail mix or granola bars, in advance so they're available when you need them.

Maintaining a Healthy and Balanced Diet

In addition to planning and preparing healthy meals, there are several other strategies you can use to maintain a healthy and balanced diet over the long term. These include:

- Making time for regular physical activity, such as going for a walk, doing yoga, or lifting weights.

- Staying hydrated by drinking plenty of water throughout the day.

- Avoiding sugary drinks and high-calorie snacks, such as candy, cookies, and chips.

- Limiting your alcohol intake, or avoiding it altogether if possible.

- Seeking support from friends, family, or a professional nutritionist if needed.

It's also important to be flexible and allow yourself some leeway in your diet. If you indulge in a treat every once in a while, that's okay! Just make sure to balance it out with healthy food choices and physical activity the rest of the time.

In conclusion, creating a sustainable and balanced diet is a journey, not a destination. By planning and preparing healthy meals, and implementing strategies to maintain a healthy diet, you can take control of your health and feel confident in your food choices. Remember, there's no one-size-fits-all approach to diet, so it's important to find what works for you and your lifestyle. With these tips, you'll be on your way to creating a sustainable and balanced diet that will help you feel your best for years to come.

Chapter 14: Overcoming Diet Fads and Quick Fixes

In recent years, the diet industry has been plagued by an abundance of fad diets and quick fixes, all promising miraculous results in a short amount of time. From the low-carb craze to the juice cleanses, these diets have caused many people to become frustrated and disillusioned with their weight loss journeys. The truth is, most of these diets are not sustainable, and even when they produce temporary results, the weight is often regained once the person returns to their normal eating habits.

The problem with fad diets and quick fixes is that they often focus on eliminating entire food groups or drastically reducing calorie intake, which can have a negative impact on overall health. Additionally, these diets often promise unrealistic results and do not take into account the individual needs and goals of each person. As a result, they are often difficult to stick to and can lead to feelings of deprivation and failure.

So how can you overcome the lure of fad diets and quick fixes? The key is to focus on creating a healthy, balanced diet that you can maintain over the long term. This means finding a diet that works for you, and not simply jumping on the latest diet trend.

To start, it is important to understand your individual needs and goals. This includes taking into account your age, gender, activity level, and any health conditions you may have. Once you have a clear understanding of your needs, you can then start to create a balanced diet that provides the nutrients your body needs to thrive.

When it comes to creating a balanced diet, it is important to include a variety of foods from all food groups, including whole grains, lean proteins, healthy fats, and plenty of fruits and vegetables. By eating a variety of foods, you will ensure that your body receives all the essential nutrients it needs to function properly.

It is also important to focus on portion control and to eat only until you are satisfied, rather than overeating. This can be accomplished by using smaller plates and practicing mindful eating techniques, such as paying attention to your food and avoiding distractions while eating.

Another key aspect of creating a sustainable and balanced diet is finding healthy and tasty ways to prepare and enjoy your food. Experimenting with different recipes, cooking methods, and seasonings can help you find new and exciting ways to enjoy healthy, nutritious meals.

Finally, it is important to be patient and persistent in your efforts to create a healthy and balanced diet. It may take some time to find the right combination of foods and meals that work for you, but with patience and persistence, you will eventually find a diet that you can stick to and enjoy over the long term.

In conclusion, the key to overcoming fad diets and quick fixes is to focus on creating a sustainable and balanced diet that works for you. By taking into account your individual needs and goals, and by finding healthy and tasty ways to prepare and enjoy your food, you can achieve your weight loss goals and enjoy a healthier, happier life.

Chapter 15: Staying Healthy and Achieving Your Diet Goals

The journey to a healthier lifestyle through diet can be a challenging one, but with the right tools and mindset, it can also be an incredibly rewarding one. Whether you are just starting out or have been following a specific diet for some time, it is important to understand the steps you can take to stay healthy and achieve your diet goals.

One of the key factors in staying healthy and reaching your diet goals is motivation. It can be easy to lose steam and slip back into old habits, but by setting clear and achievable goals, you can stay motivated and on track. Consider writing down your goals and keeping them visible, such as in a journal or on a whiteboard, so you can see your progress and stay focused on what you want to achieve.

Another important factor in maintaining a healthy and balanced diet is avoiding common pitfalls. One of the most common obstacles is the temptation to turn to quick fixes or fad diets. These types of diets may promise rapid weight loss, but they are often not sustainable, and can even be harmful to your health. Instead, focus on adopting a balanced and healthy diet that includes a variety of foods from all food groups.

In addition to avoiding common pitfalls, it is also important to be mindful of portion sizes and avoid overeating. Try to eat slowly, and listen to your body when it tells you that you are full. Additionally, make sure to stay hydrated by drinking plenty of water throughout the day.

It is also important to maintain a healthy and balanced lifestyle, which includes exercise and other physical activity. Regular exercise has numerous benefits, including improved physical health, increased energy, and reduced stress. When it comes to diet, remember that it is not just about what you eat, but also about how you live.

In conclusion, finding the right diet for you and maintaining a healthy and balanced lifestyle can be challenging, but with the right tools and mindset, it is an achievable goal. By staying motivated, avoiding common pitfalls, and maintaining a balanced lifestyle, you can achieve your diet goals and enjoy a healthier and happier life. Remember that a healthy and balanced diet is an important part of a healthy and balanced lifestyle, and by making.

In conclusion, this book has provided an in-depth analysis of the various popular diets that are currently available, including their history, the scientific evidence behind them, and the potential benefits and drawbacks of each one. Throughout the book, we have discussed the importance of a healthy and balanced diet, and provided practical advice for readers who are looking to find the right diet for them, create a sustainable and balanced diet, and overcome the lure of fad diets and quick fixes.

In the final chapter, we emphasized the importance of staying healthy and achieving your diet goals, and provided practical tips on how to do so. Whether you are looking to lose weight, improve your overall health, or simply maintain a healthy and balanced lifestyle, the key is to make informed decisions about your diet, and to stick to a healthy and balanced diet over the long term.

In the end, we hope that this book has provided you with the information and inspiration you need to make the most of your health and well-being. Whether you are just starting out on your journey to a healthier lifestyle, or you are already well on your way, we wish you all the best in your efforts to achieve your goals. So go ahead and take control of your health and well-being, and make the most of the opportunities that a healthy and balanced diet has to offer!